I0113793

The Small Birds and the Big Bully Snake

WRITTEN BY:
DR. ANISH BABU ZACHARIA

ILLUSTRATED BY:
AJIMON M.M

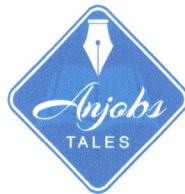

Anjobs TALES

DISCLAIMER

The Small Birds and the Big Bully Snakes

Copyrights Reserved © 2021 – Dr. Anish Babu Zacharia

No part of this Book can be transmitted or reproduced in any form including print, electronic, photocopying, scanning, mechanical or recording without prior written permission from the author.

The author takes no charge of the opinion that any of the third-party or unrelated individuals have. If the content inculcated in the publication becomes obsolete due to technical reasons or whatsoever, the author or the publication house are entitled to no blames.
All of the events indicated in the book are the result of personal experience and observation of the person(s) involved in formulating the book and bringing it into the form it is in, today.

All the content used in this book belongs solely to the author. However, there may be mistakes in typography or content. Also, this Book provides information only up to the publishing date. Therefore, this Book should be used as a guide and not as the ultimate source.

Dedication

This book is dedicated in memory of my loving mother who always encouraged me to strive higher.

About the Author

Dr. Anish Babu Zacharia holds a Doctorate Degree in Consumer Neuroscience from SP Jain School Of Global Business, Sydney, a MS Degree in Electrical Engineering from California State University, Long Beach; a MBA degree from Lucas Graduate School of Business, San Jose State University, California; a B.Tech degree in Electronics and Telecommunication from TKM College of Engineering, India; and Honors Diploma in Computer Networking from NIIT, India. He is an entrepreneur who always tries to find time from his busy work life to write stories.

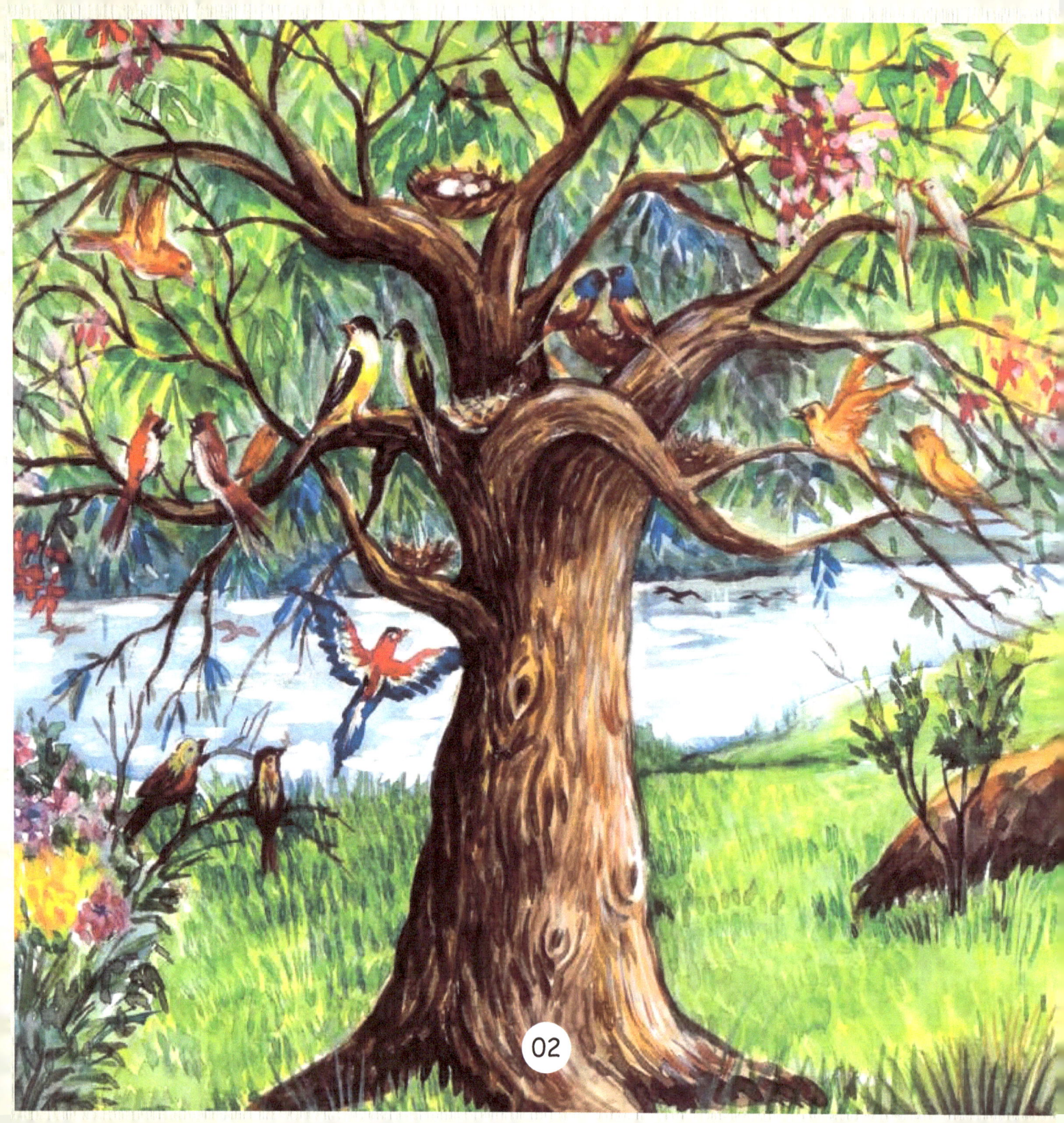

02

Once upon a time, on a big tree covered with lots of colorful flowers and leaves there lived a flock of small birds. The tree was surrounded by beautiful gardens and a beautiful river with clean flowing water.

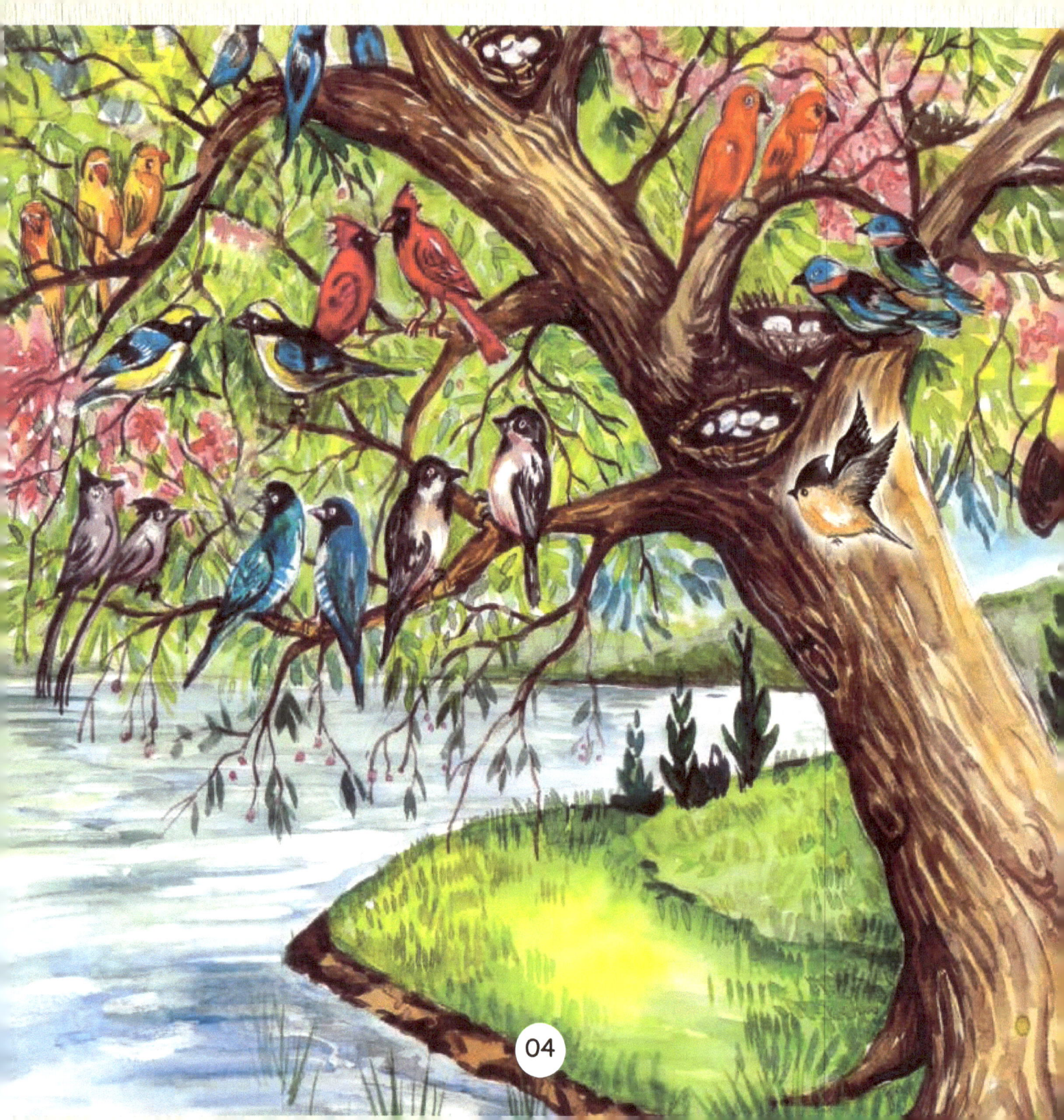

The tree housed a lot of nests for different birds with different shapes and colors. The birds' families enjoyed their beautiful homes in the tree and enjoyed their happy lives. On the tree one could see the bird chicks and fledglings playing and singing all day with their friends with a cacophony of melodious symphonies. The tree was always surrounded by beautifully colored birds flying around.

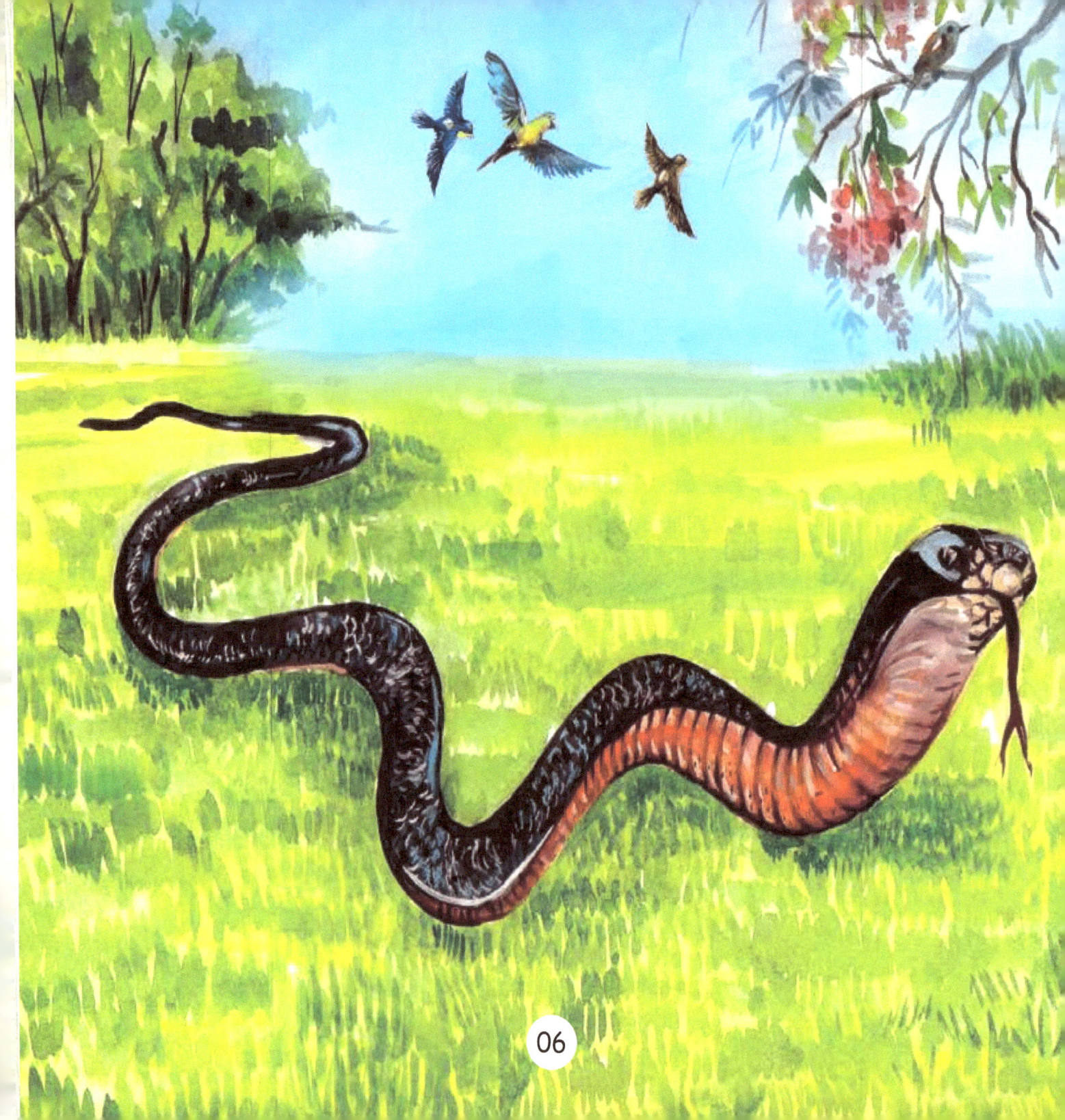

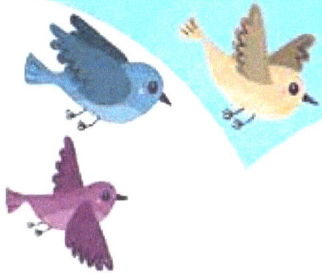

One day, a big black snake with a red belly was crawling through the gardens near the tree. As the snake was passing by the tree, he heard the sounds of the birds on the tree.

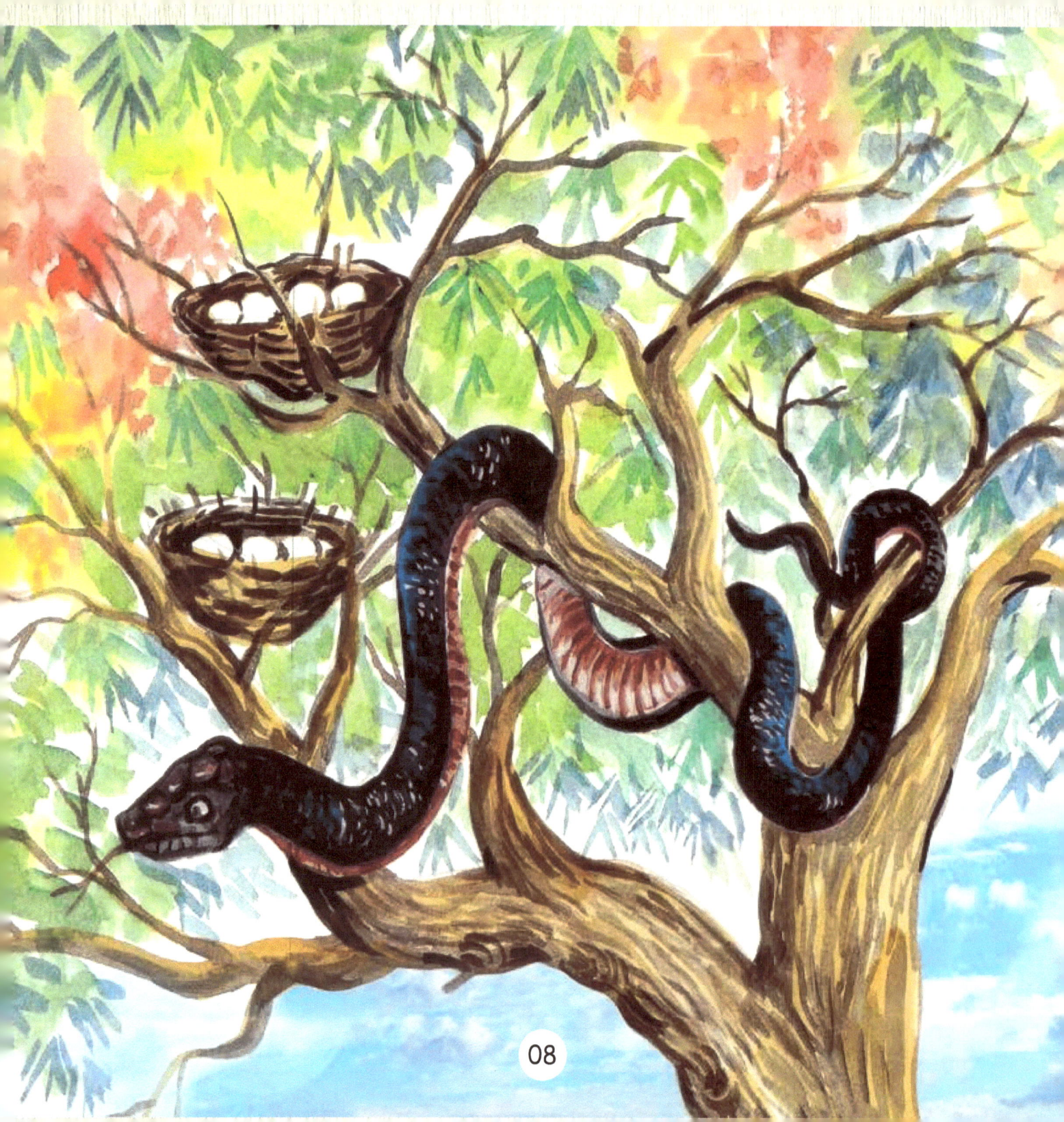

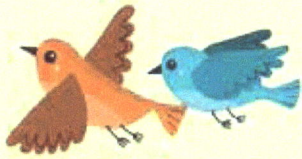

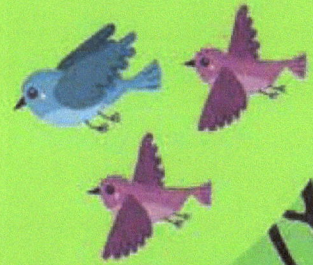

Intrigued with the sounds, the snake moved serpentinely up the tree to see it teeming with a large number of nests which housed a lot of birds and eggs. He was delighted to see so many birds and eggs. The snake thought about the number of days he was going to feast deliciously.

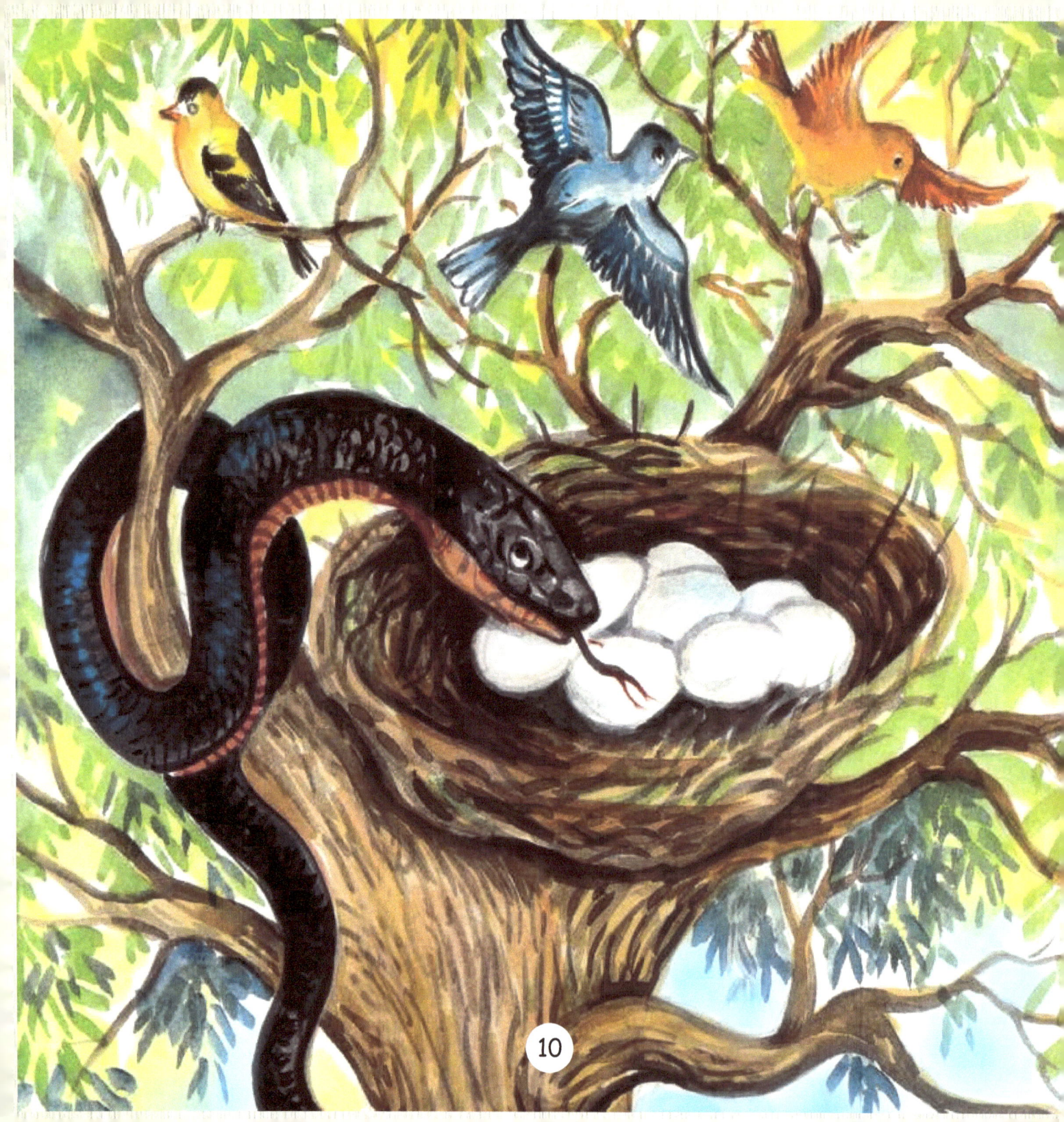

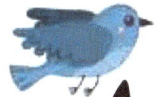

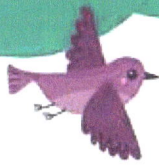

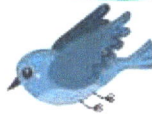

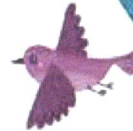

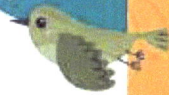

As the snake glided further up the tree and got closer to the birds, the birds alarmed each other by squawking loudly. Suddenly all the birds flew away from the nests leaving the eggs behind.

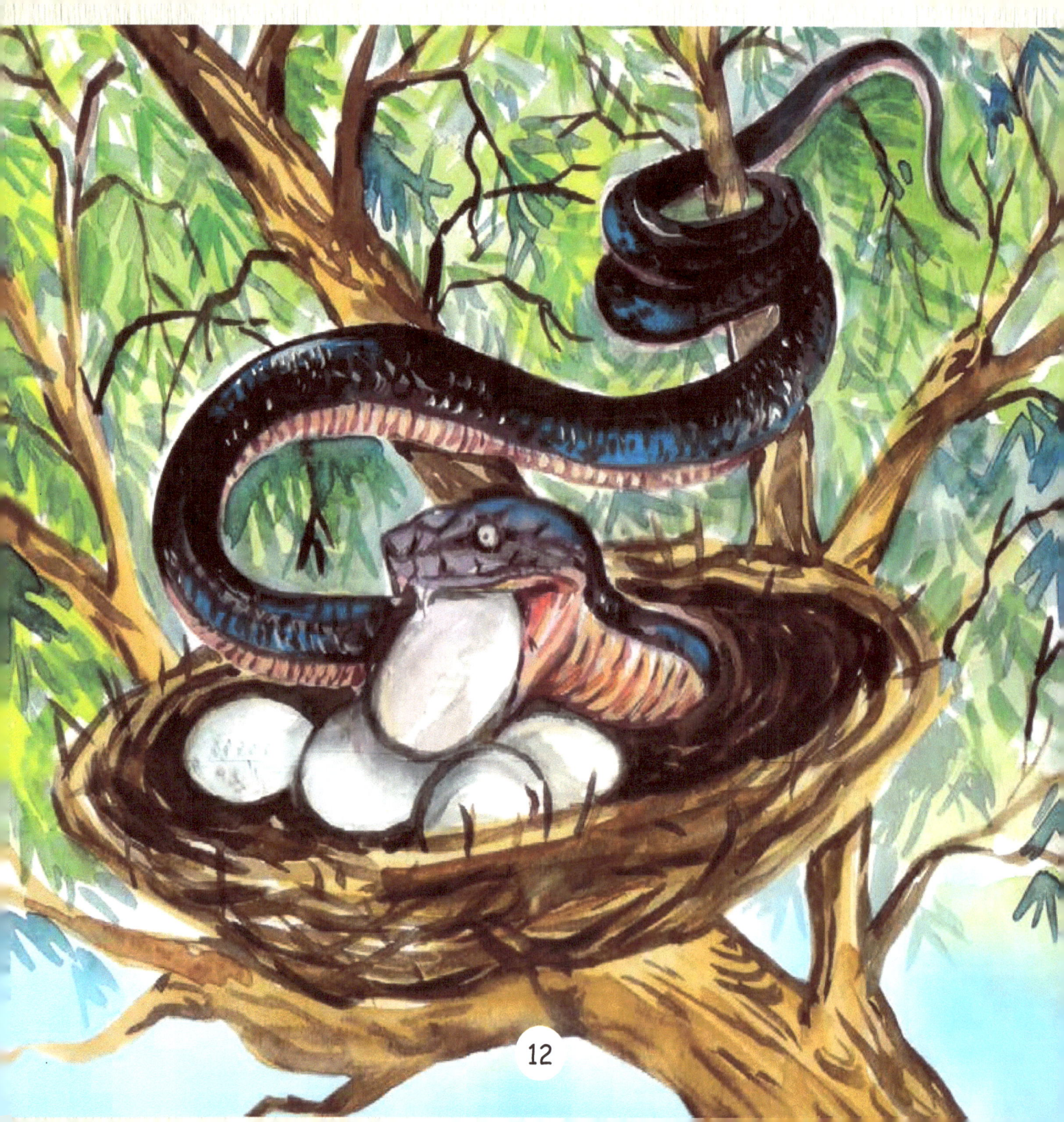

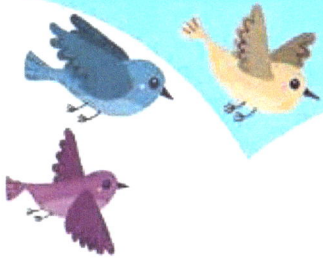

The snake delightedly swallowed few eggs and reminded the birds that he would come whenever he pleased and would take more eggs. He also warned them sternly that it would be best to obey him, as he was bigger and stronger than the small birds.

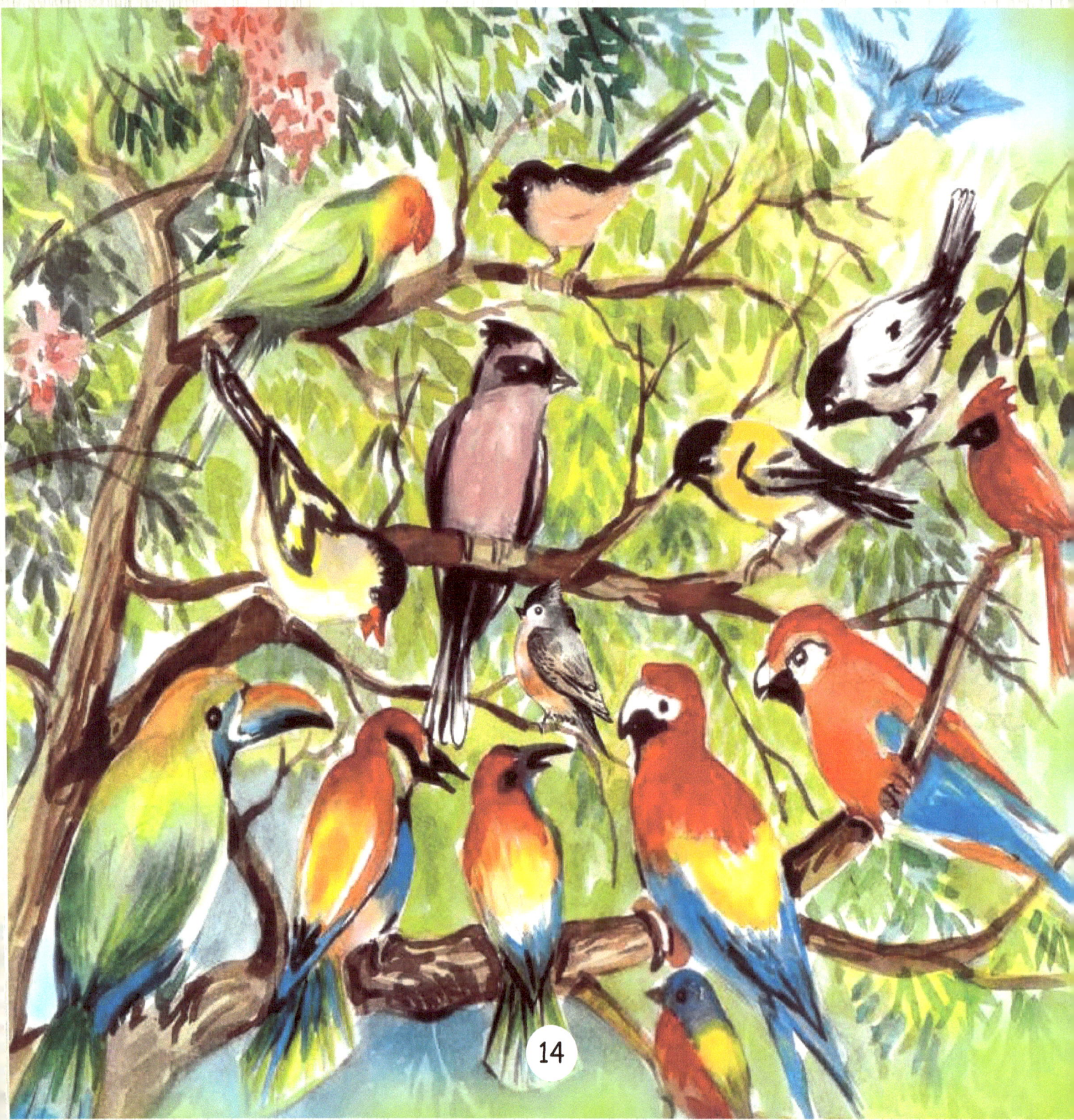

14

After this, all birds became sad and frightened. They got together and tried to come up with plans to overcome the snake, but was unsuccessful to come with a strong plan. The snake came again as he pleased a few more times and took most of the birds' eggs. Seeing this, birds were frightened to lay more eggs as the snake would come and take them away.

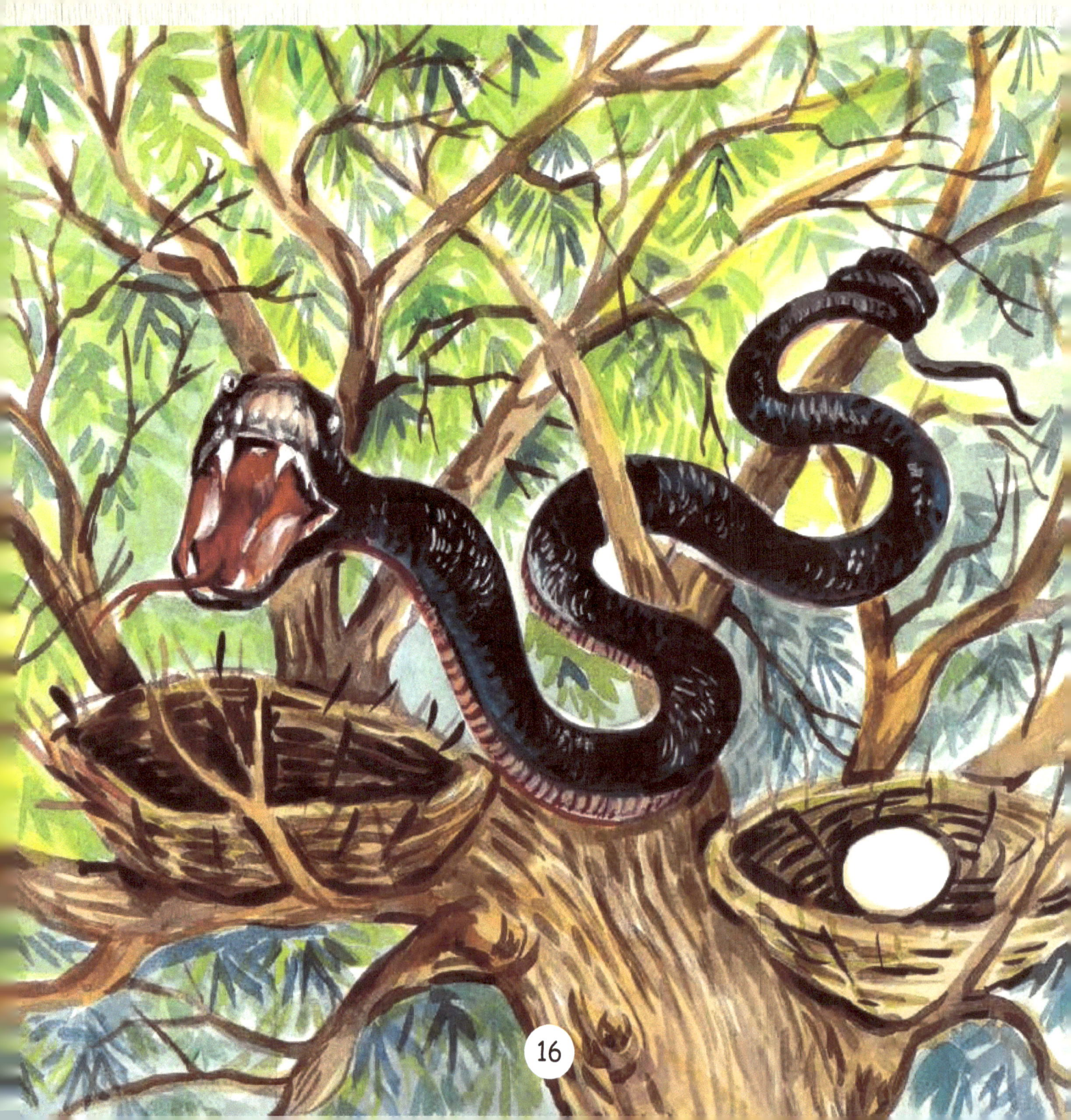

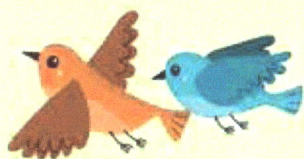

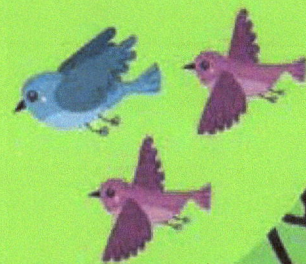

When the snake came again, he saw that the number of eggs were becoming fewer each time he came. Perturbed at having his sustenance dwindling, he threatened the birds that if there were no more eggs he would start catching and eating the birds.

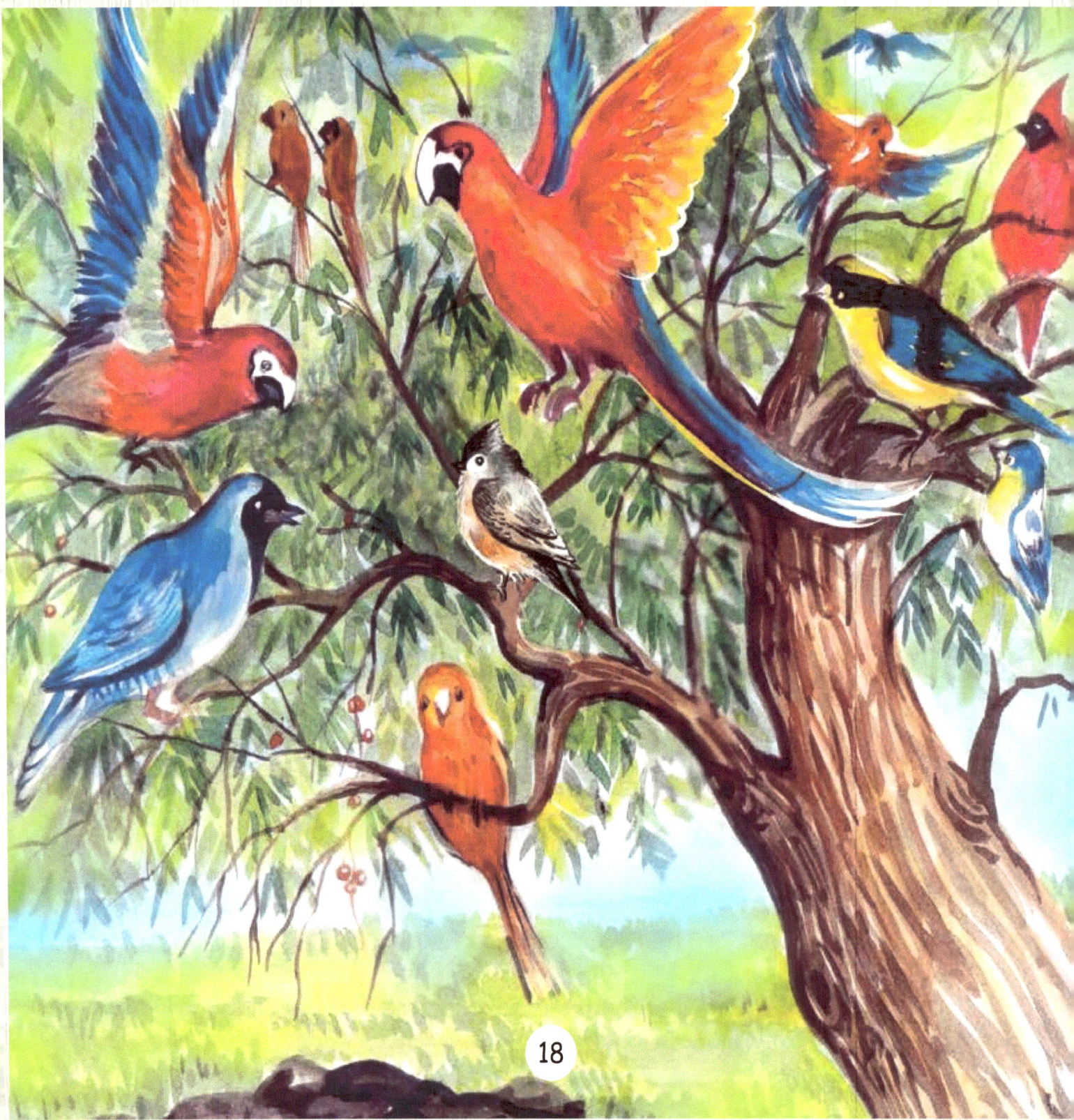

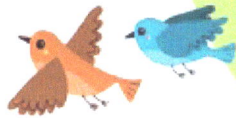

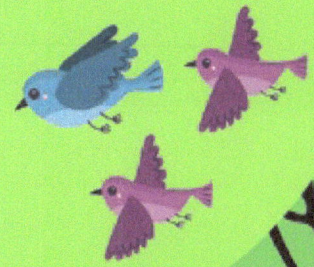

After the snake left the birds started
feeling more frightened. They all got together
again to decide what to do for their future. Some birds
suggested to leave the tree forever and move to a new
tree, while some birds came up with plan of attacking the
snake as a flock altogether at one time. But a small bird
who was listening to all the different plans came to the
front and said "Can I say a plan". On hearing this the
bigger birds started scolding the small bird and said this
is not the time for telling stories. But undeterred, the
small bird did not let others stop him and he started
yelling louder with his plans. The other birds became
quieter and started listening.

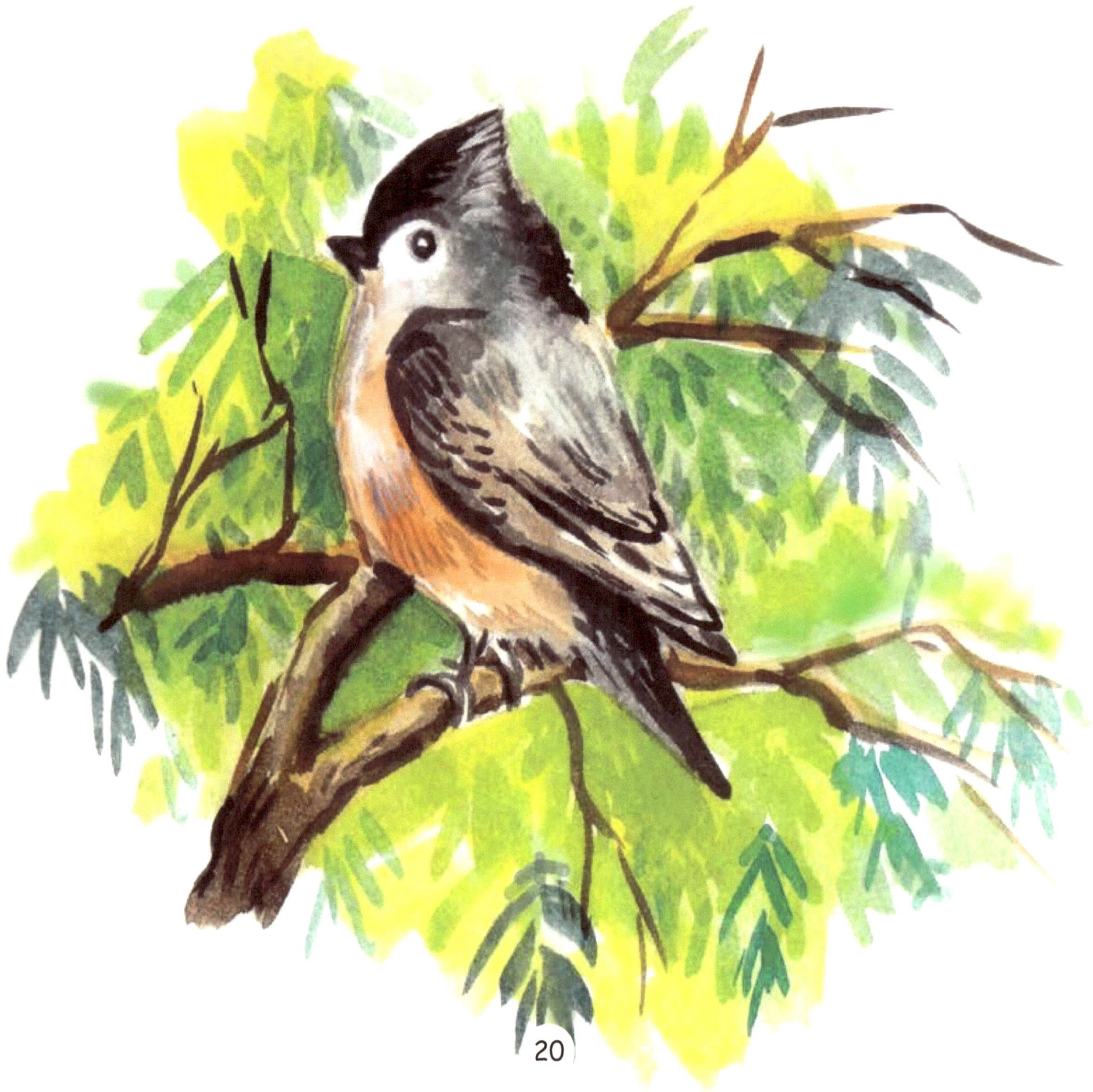

The small bird said the snake knew their weakness of small size and the birds would fly away from the nest when the snake scared them. So, the same way they should also know the weakness of the snake. The other birds became more curious and paid more attention to what the small bird said. He said, "Have you noticed that the snake swallows the eggs and never uses his teeth. After swallowing the eggs, he goes to some place where he can rest and eat its food comfortably. This is our opportunity and the snake's weakness." This got the other birds thinking. They listened with a surprised and confused look.

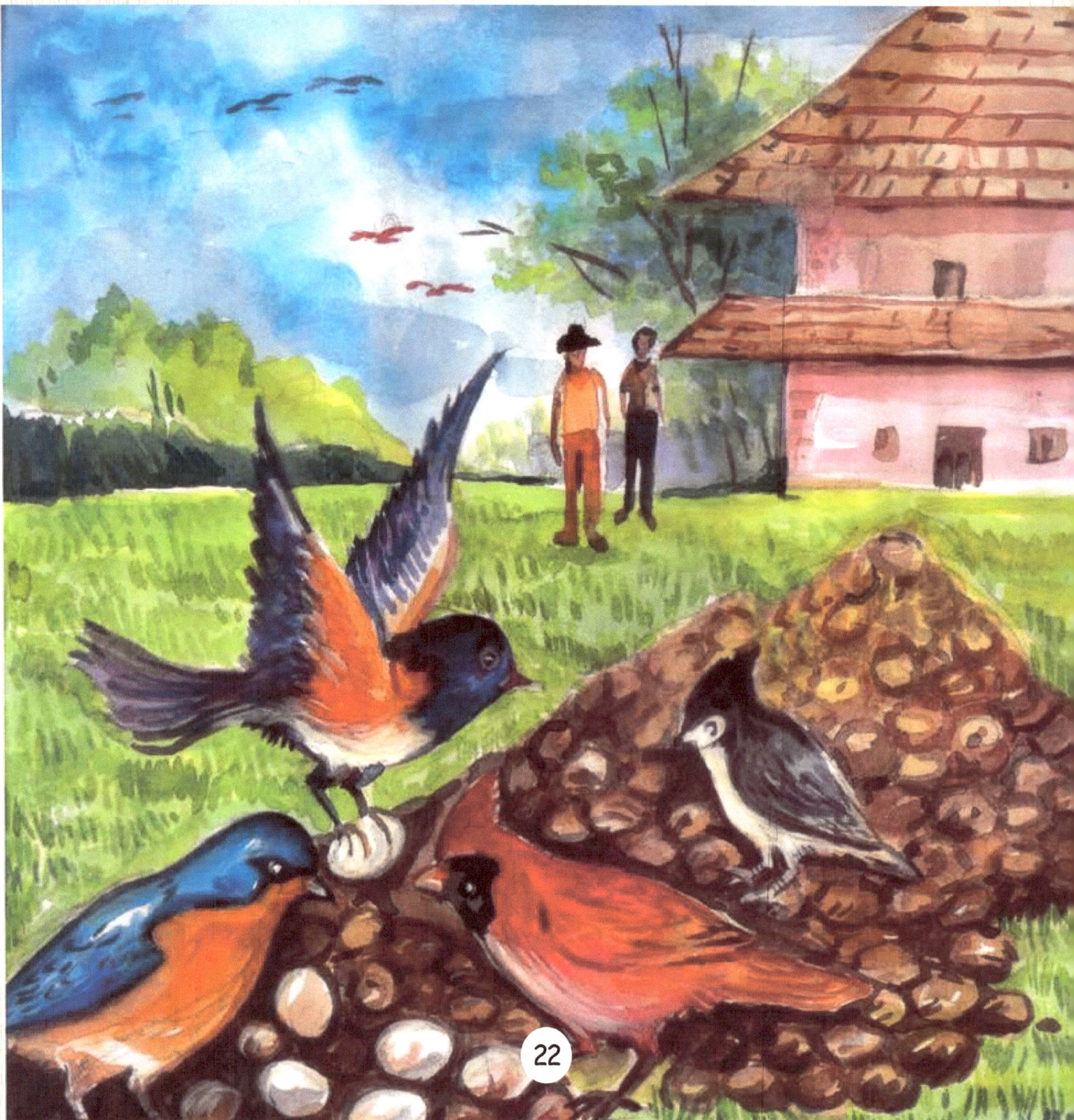

22

The small bird started laying out his plan. He explained that in order to get rid of the snake they had to sacrifice a few more eggs. He asked the birds to start laying eggs, and let the snake come and swallow few of these eggs. He further asked everyone to find some nice white oval shape stones which are nearly the same size of the eggs. Then place these stones in between the eggs in the nest. Since the snake always swallow the eggs, he will swallow these stones also. Once the snake swallows the stones, the stones would incapacitate the snake. All the birds thought this was a good idea and their best chance.

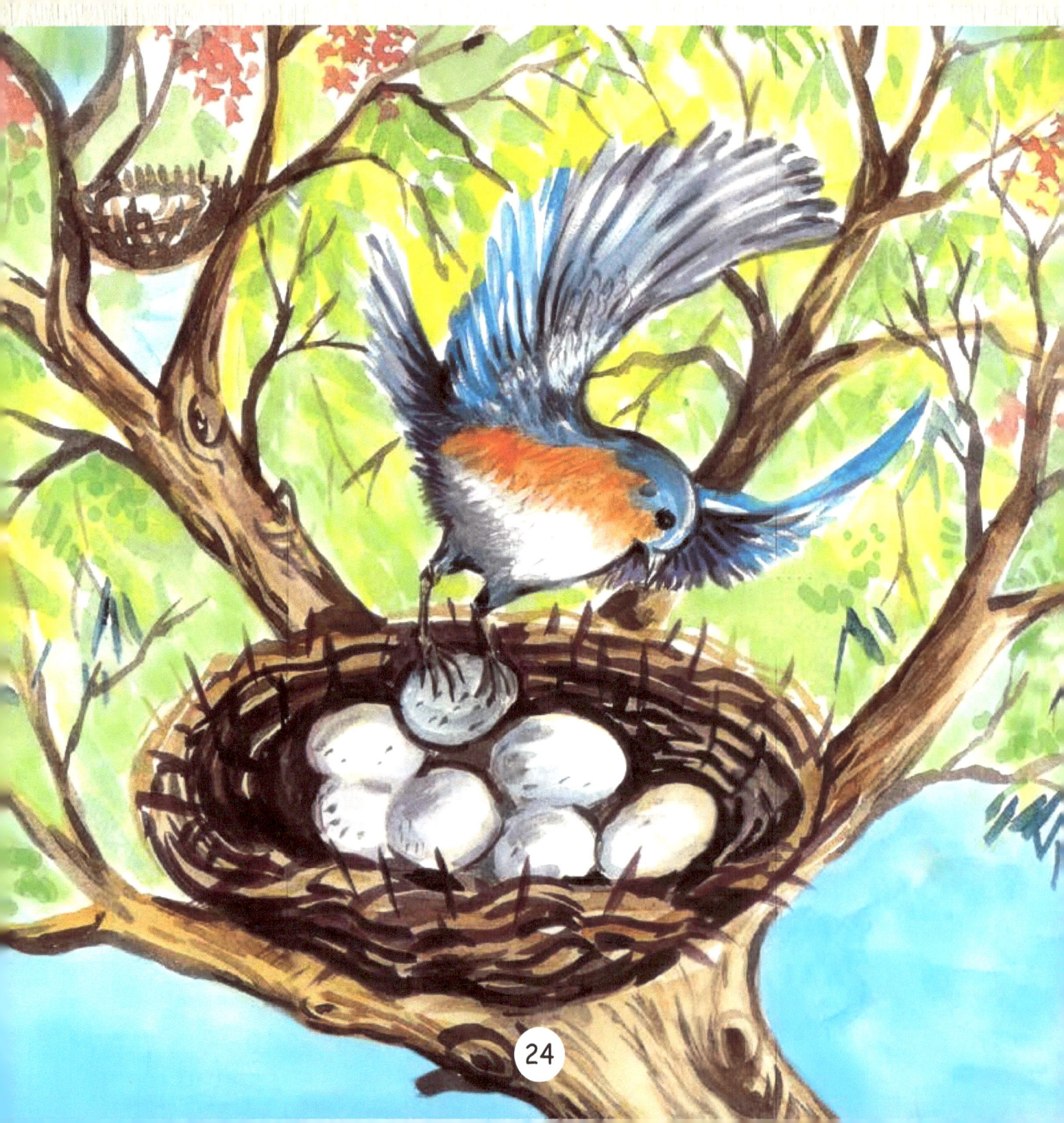

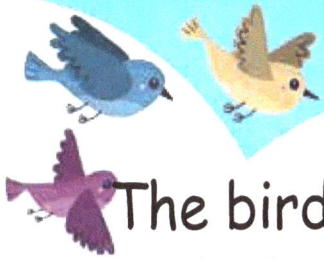

The birds flew around the neighborhood to find white oval shaped stones. Soon they were able to find few stones but the stones were heavy. So, the birds had to work together to bring the stones to their nest. They were really tired after working to bring the stone to their nests.

After few days the birds started laying eggs in their nest and hid the stones in between the eggs. The stones were placed in a such a way that no one could differentiate between the original eggs and the stones.

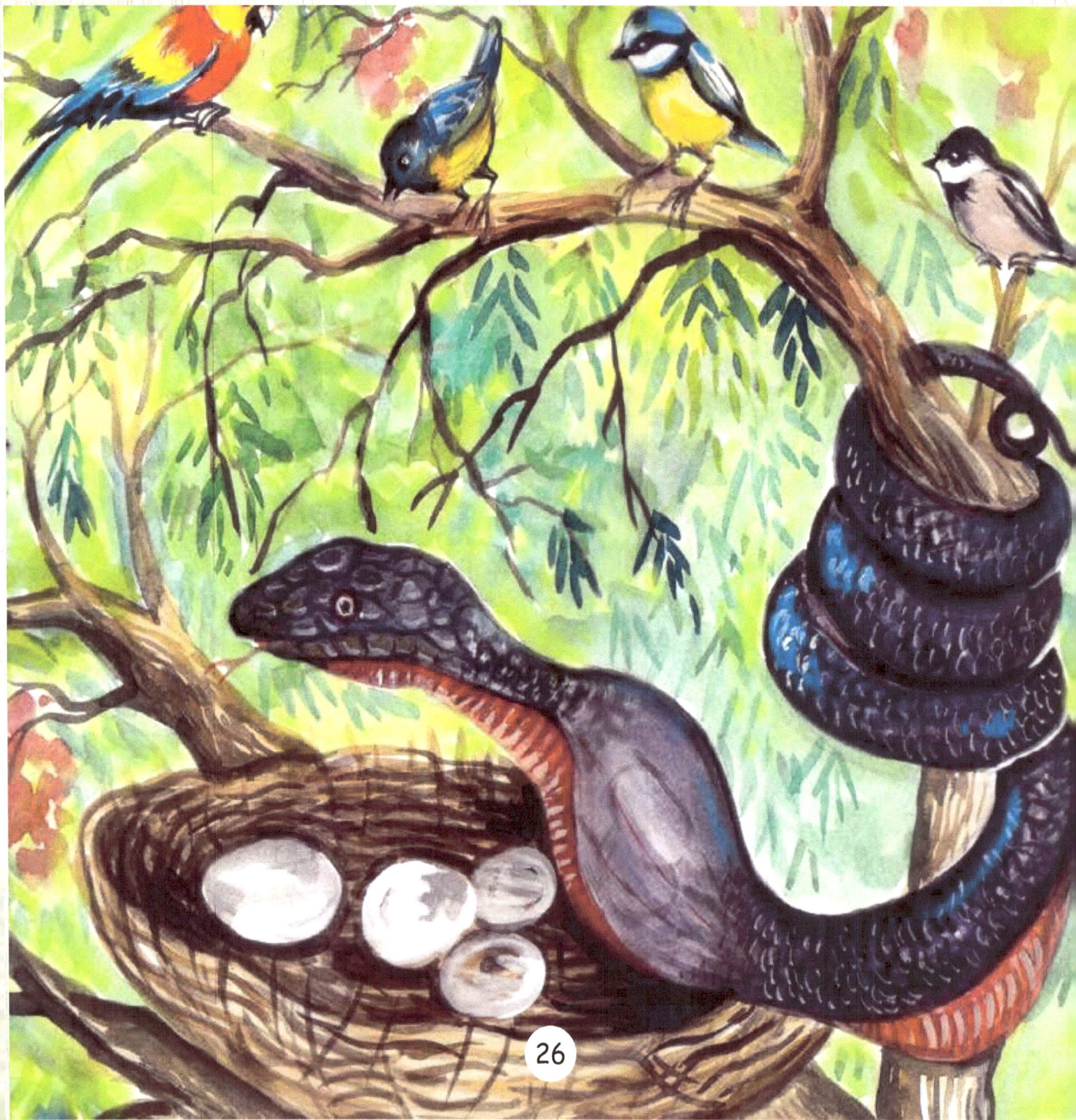

26

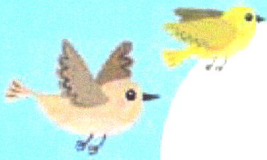

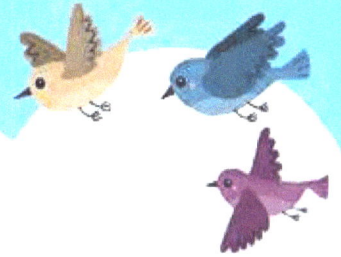

As expected after few days the snake returned. He was delighted to see so many eggs in the nest. The snake thought how mighty and strong he was, as he could coerce and bully the small birds to do what he wanted. He was so excited that he hastily went around swallowing maximum number of eggs from the nests to have a sumptuous meal.

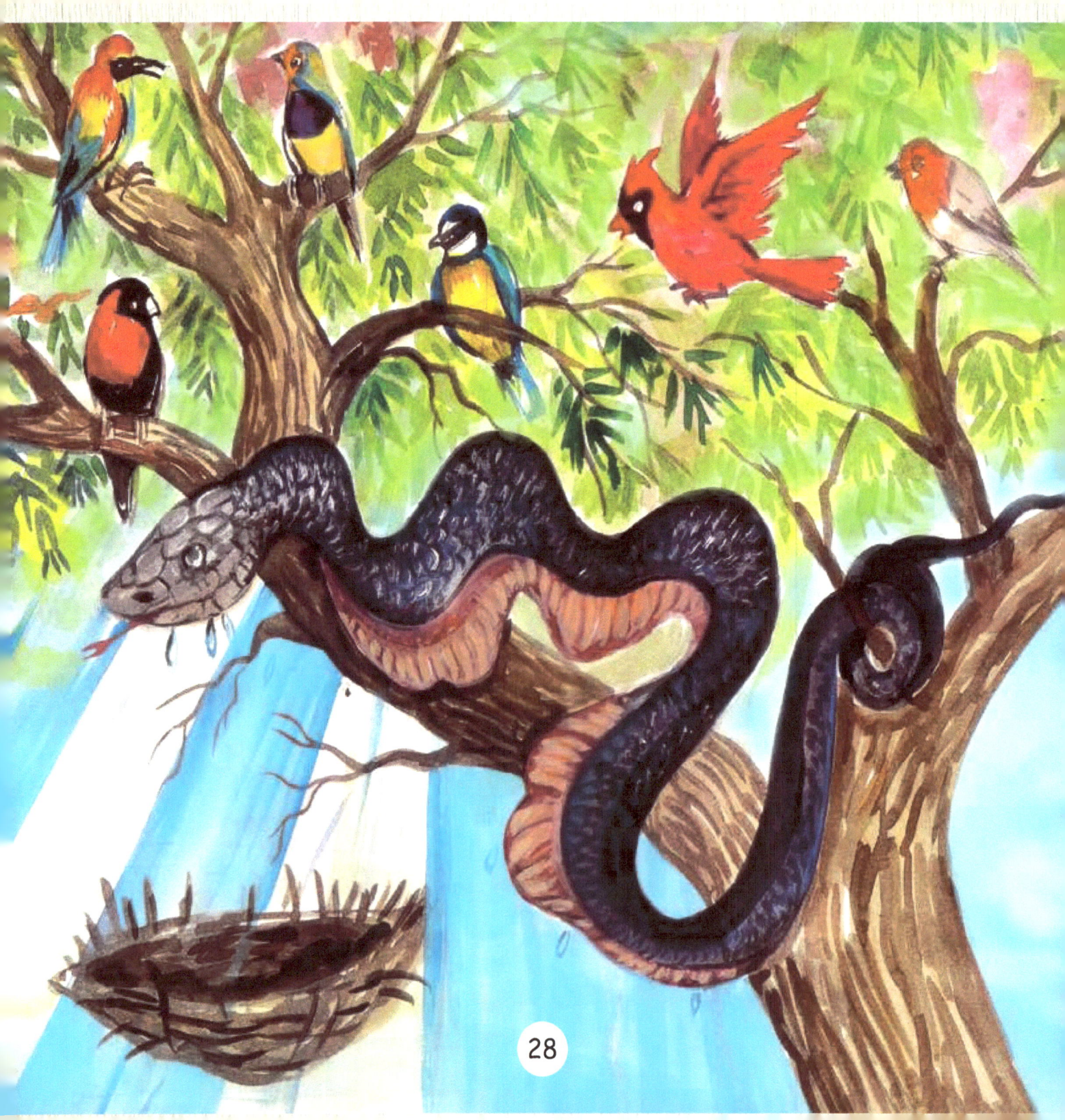

The birds kept a watch from a safe distance and was sad about losing their eggs. They tried to console each other while the snake swallowed the eggs from their nests. As the snake took more and more eggs, he also swallowed lot of stones along with the eggs. As he started moving along the tree branches, he couldn't control his balance as the heavy stones inside his body started pulling his body to different sides.

29

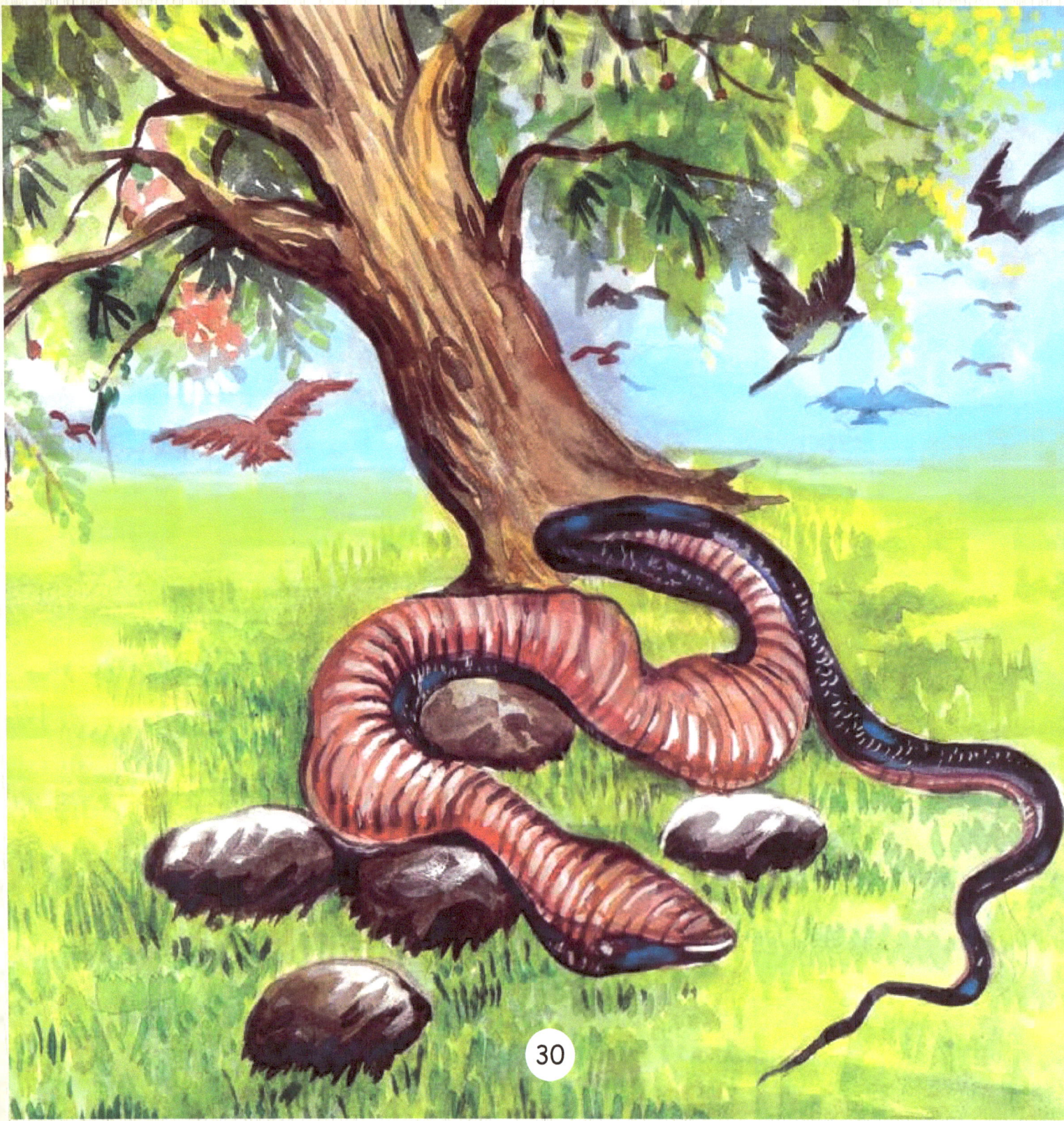

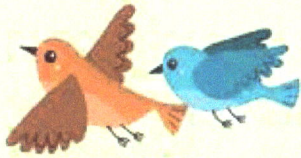

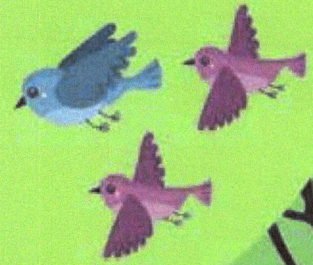

Finally, the snake lost his balance and
fell down from the tall tree.
The impact of the heavy stones
and the high fall killed
the snake.

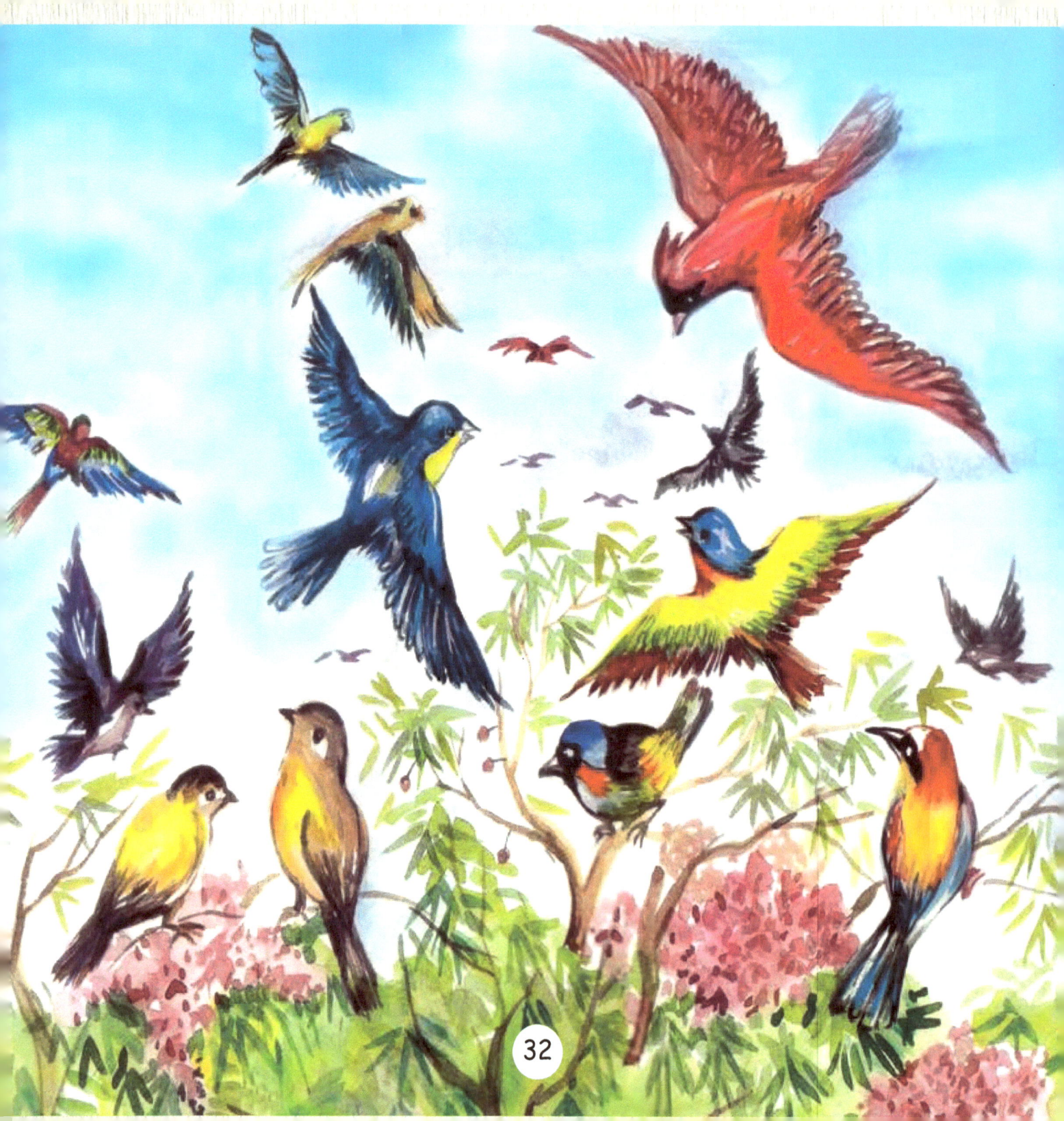

32

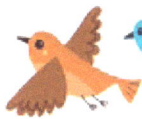

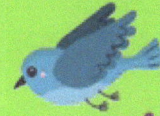

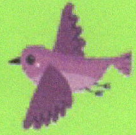

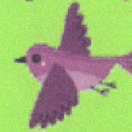

On seeing this, all birds started
flying around with glee and
singing with utmost untold joy.
They have never been so
happy in their life.

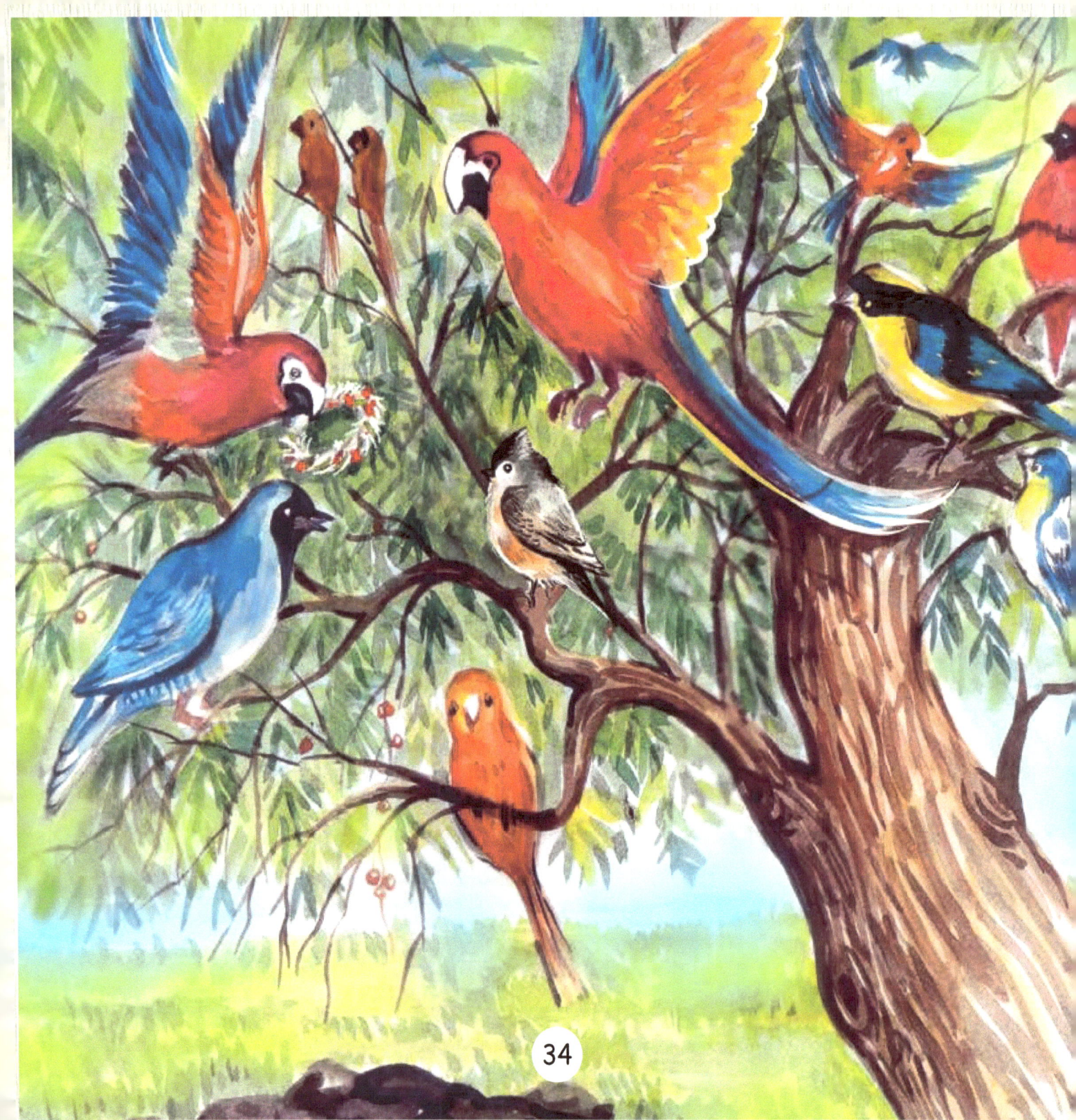

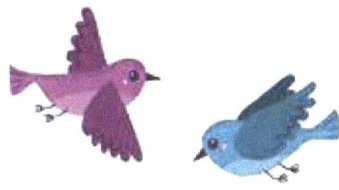
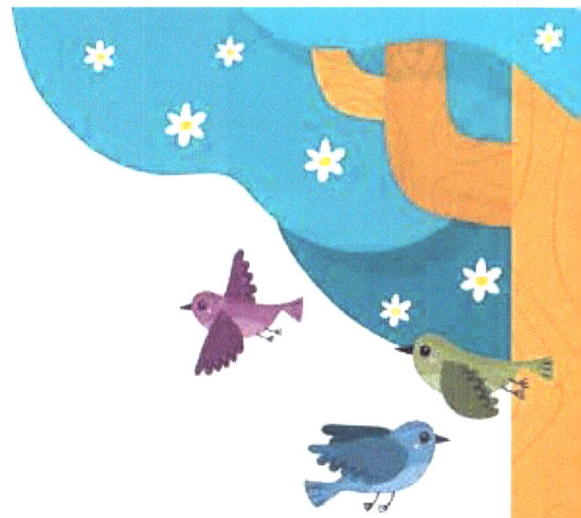

They were very thankful to the small bird
for his unthinkable plan and promised
the small bird that they would always
listen to what the small
birds have to say.

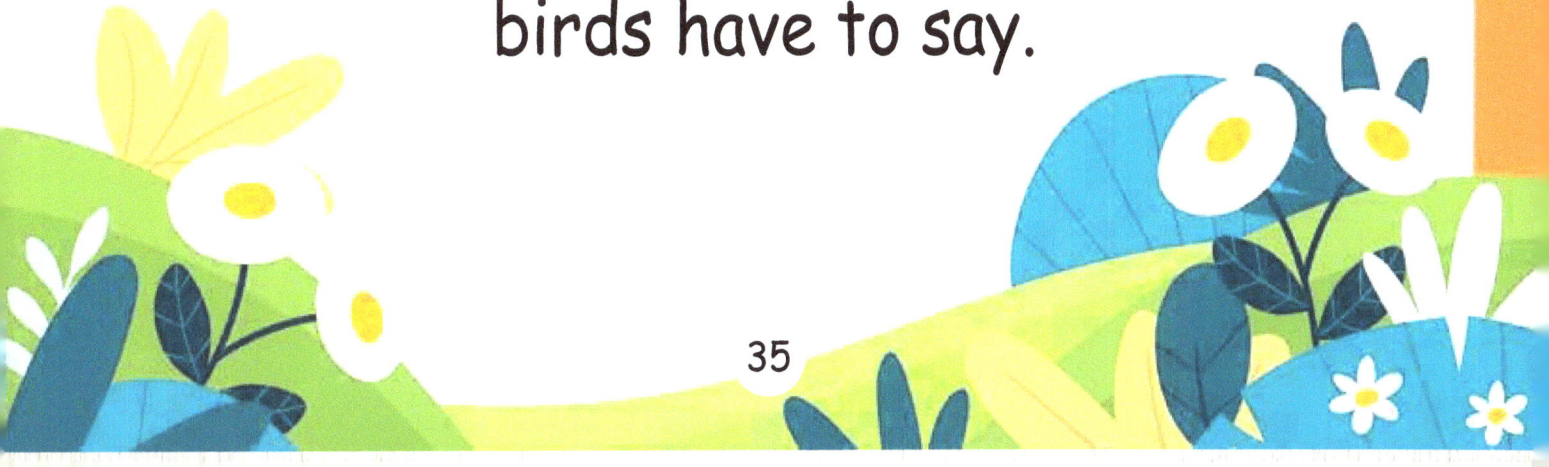

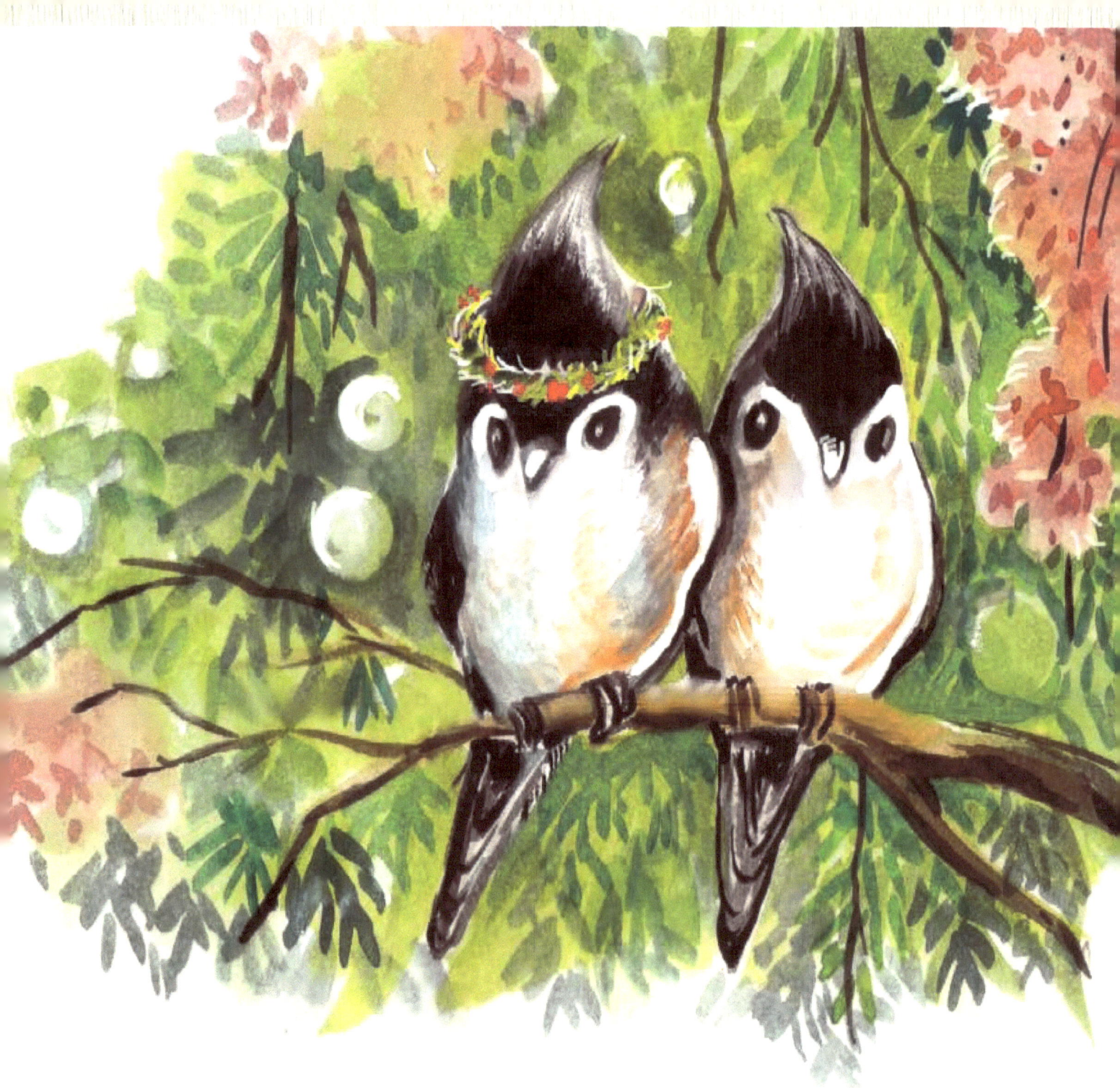

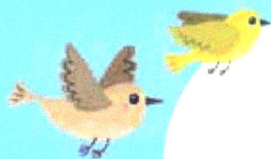

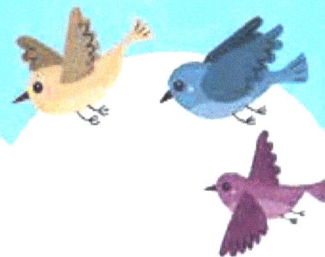

The moral of the story is that any bully or a strong creature cannot remain strong or mighty every time. They too have weakness and if this weakness is understood by their smaller or weaker victims, then these victims can overcome the mighty bullies once and forever. The weak and the meek can stand tall yet again.

Summary

Through this book 'The Small Birds and the Big Bully Snake', the author, Dr. Anish Babu Zacharia takes one into the stunning world of small birds by way of a captivating story and truly colorful pictures. This gorgeous world of birds, exactly where the birds enjoy singing and playing every single day comes to an unexpected halt when a huge snake discovers their home and begin threatening and bullying them into obeying him. But even though the little birds were no match against the snake, they come up with a cunning way to defeat the snake. These seemingly insignificant birds succeed in their plan and surprise everyone who doubted the defeat of the snake in the hands of the tiny birds.

'The Small Birds and the Big Bully Snake', tries to convey and create confidence among the young readers that no matter how strong or mighty the bully or perhaps the enemy is, all of them have a weakness and if you are able to discover that weakness, you are able to overcome your enemy or bully.

Acknowledgements

First and foremost, I would like to thank God for his never-ending grace, mercy and his blessings showered on me to write stories for children.

Next, I would like to thank my first critics – my two daughters Alisha and Angelin; and my nephew Aaron for whom I started writing these stories. I thank my loving and supporting father, my loving wife, my brother and my sister-in-law for the all the support and encouragement extended towards me in coming out with this book.

THE END

www.ingramcontent.com/pod-product-compliance
Lightning Source LLC
Chambersburg PA
CBHW060859270326
41935CB00003B/37